RENAL DIET
COOKBOOK FOR BEGINNERS

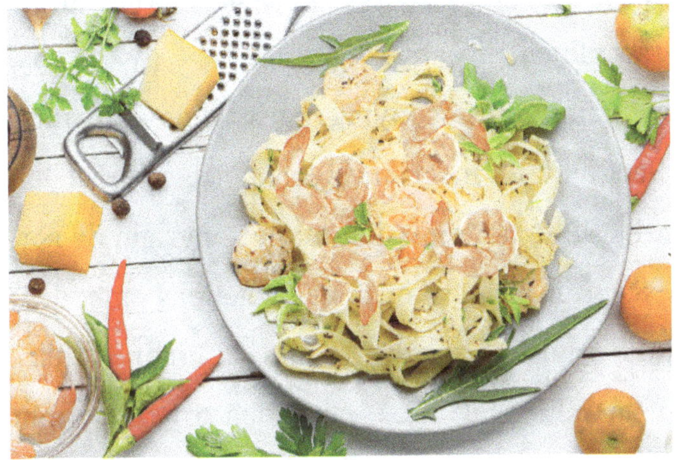

Caring for Your Kidneys with Flavorful Dishes and Practical Guidance

Dr. Jaclyn N. Anderson

Table of Contents

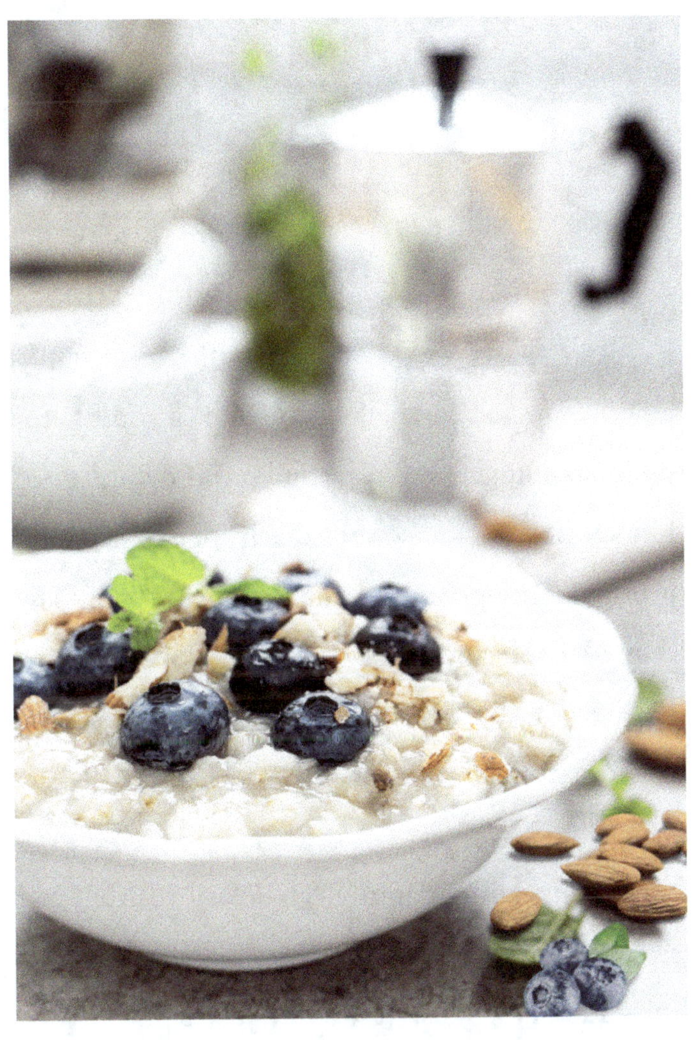

INTRODUCTION

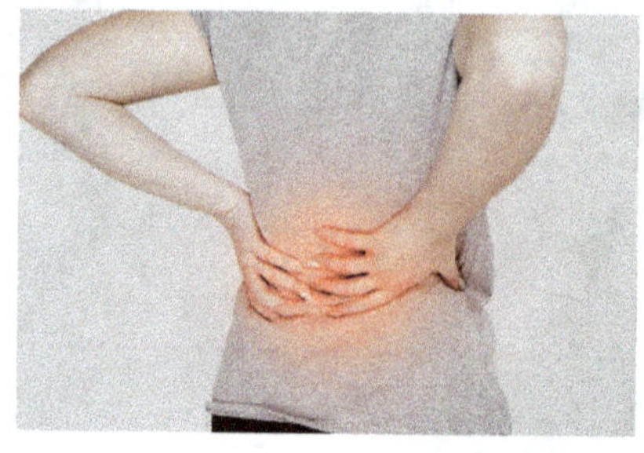 Isabella's journey with the renal diet began with uncertainty and a quest for understanding. Facing the complexities of kidney health, she sought clarity, guidance, and a practical approach to managing her diet. The "Renal Diet Cookbook for Beginners" became her beacon, a trove of knowledge, and a source of culinary inspiration.

Struggling with adapting to dietary restrictions, Isabella found solace in the cookbook's introductory pages. It wasn't just a list of dos and don'ts; it was a supportive hand guiding her through the nuances of a renal diet. Exploring the recipes, she discovered a vibrant world of flavors and nourishing ingredients specifically tailored for kidney health. From the comforting embrace of a homemade low-sodium soup to the colorful allure of a berry parfait, each recipe painted a canvas of hope and possibility.

As Isabella delved into the chapters, she found not just meals but a renewed sense of control and empowerment over her health. The cookbook's nutritional insights and explanations were a roadmap, clarifying the impact of her dietary choices on her well-being. The recipes were not just culinary creations; they were a path to wellness and vitality.

Guided by the cookbook, Isabella embarked on a journey of exploration, experimentation, and triumph. It was more than a collection of recipes; it became her faithful companion, offering support and encouragement through her dietary transformation. The cookbook's approach was not just about food; it was a mindful and compassionate philosophy that fostered her understanding of a kidney-healthy lifestyle.

Now, as Isabella shares her story, she hopes to inspire others starting their own renal diet journey. She found in this cookbook not just a guide, but a narrative of resilience, empowerment, and a testament to the transformative power of embracing a kidney-healthy diet. This introductory story encapsulates not just her journey but the promise of hope and healing for all who seek a path to improved well-being through the nurturing embrace of a renal diet.

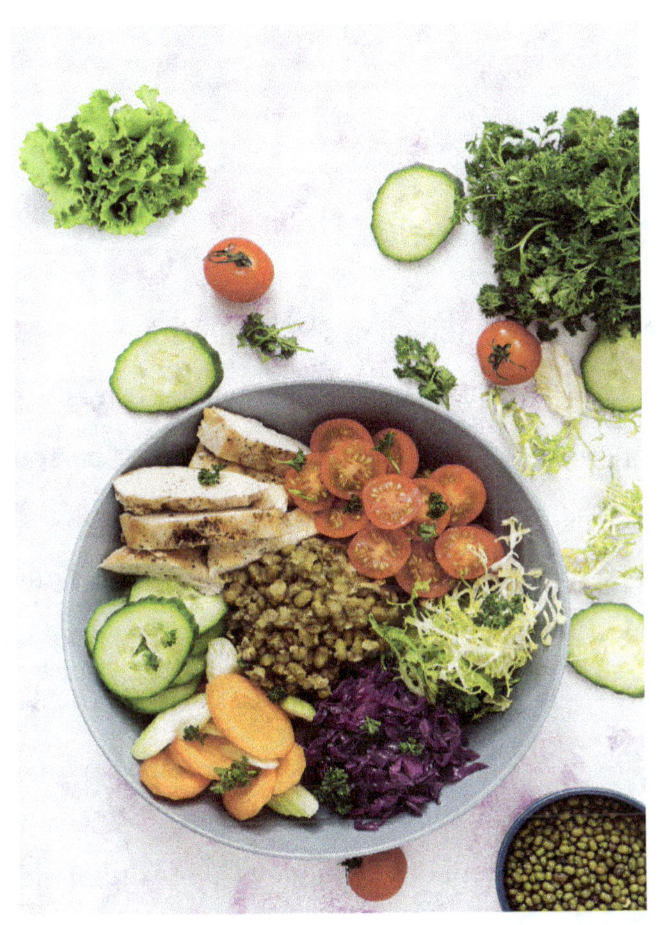

CHAPTER 1:

UNDERSTANDING KIDNEY HEALTH

Benefits of a Renal Diet

A kidney-friendly diet, sometimes referred to as a renal diet, is one that is created expressly to support and advance kidney health. For persons with kidney illness or who are at risk of developing kidney problems, this specific diet has many advantages. These are the principal advantages of a renal diet:

1. **Manage Kidney Function:** By easing the strain on the kidneys, a renal diet aids in the management of kidney function. It makes the bloodstream less likely to build up with wastes and poisons, which helps the kidneys work more effectively.

2. **Control Blood Pressure:** One of the most frequent side effects of renal illness is high blood pressure. Reduced sodium consumption is a common component of a renal diet, which helps control blood pressure and lowers the risk of cardiac problems.

3. **Reduce Fluid Retention:** Fluid retention can be brought on by kidney disease. A renal diet limits excessive fluid intake, assisting in the prevention of edema and maintaining a healthy fluid balance in the body.

4. **Controlling Electrolyte Levels:** The kidneys control electrolytes like calcium, phosphorus, and potassium. These electrolytes are carefully regulated by a renal diet, minimizing imbalances that could be detrimental to bone and heart health.

5. **Avoid Protein Buildup:** A diet high in protein might put a burden on the kidneys. A renal diet typically contains moderate amounts of high-quality protein sources to avoid overtaxing the kidneys while preventing waste product buildup.

6. **Reduce Uremic Symptoms:** A renal diet can help with uremia-related symptoms such weariness, nausea, and appetite loss. These signs are reduced by reducing waste product buildup.

7. **Maintain Bone Health:** Because of calcium and phosphorus imbalances caused by kidney illness, bones can become brittle. These minerals are kept at the proper levels to support bone health by the renal diet.

8. **Improve Overall Nutrition:** An emphasis on fresh fruits, vegetables, lean proteins, and whole grains helps to

improve overall nutrition while a renal diet restricts some nutrients. Better general health and well-being may result from this.

9. **Reduced chance of Complications:** Adopting a renal diet can reduce your chance of developing kidney disease-related complications such cardiovascular problems, anemia, and kidney failure.

10. **Enhance Quality of Life:** A renal diet can considerably improve the quality of life for those with kidney disease by controlling kidney function and reducing symptoms. They might feel better and be able to keep their freedom.

11. **Customization:** Individual demands and kidney disease stages can be taken into account when designing a renal diet. A licensed dietician or medical professional can offer individualized advice, ensuring

that the diet is suitable for each person's particular circumstances.

Kidney-Friendly Foods

For people with kidney issues, such as those who are on dialysis or have chronic kidney disease (CKD), maintaining a kidney-friendly diet is essential. Such a diet can lessen the risk of further kidney damage and assist in managing the illness. The following foods are kidney-friendly:

1. **Fruits Low in Potassium:** Choose fruits low in potassium, like apples, berries, grapes, and peaches. Your kidneys won't be overworked by these.

2. **Vegetables low in potassium:** Focus on green beans, broccoli, cabbage, and cauliflower. Compared to potatoes,

spinach, and tomatoes, they have less potassium.

3. **Lean Proteins:** Opt for lean protein sources including skinless fish, chicken, and egg whites. They contain less phosphorus, which is good for the kidneys.

4. **Low-Sodium Foods:** For the health of your kidneys, you must cut back on your sodium intake. Choose fresh or frozen foods instead of processed ones. You may manage your salt intake by cooking at home.

5. **Healthy Fats:** Include healthy fats in your diet, such as olive oil, avocados, and almonds. These fats are nutritious and good for the heart.

6. **Limit phosphorus intake:** Consume phosphorus-rich foods in moderation, such as dairy products, nuts, and seeds. If

your doctor advises using phosphate binders, follow his advice.

7. **Low-Potassium Grains:** White rice, pasta, and bread are lower in potassium than whole grains like brown rice and whole wheat bread.

8. **Spices and herbs:** Instead of salt, use spices and herbs like basil, oregano, and garlic to flavor your cuisine. You consume less salt as a result.

9. **Fluid Intake Restrictions:** Your fluid intake may need to be restricted depending on your health. Follow the recommendations for daily fluid limitations from your doctor.

10. **Portion Control:** Control portion sizes by paying attention to them. Even healthful foods, if consumed in excess, can cause problems.

11. **Diet for Dialysis Patients:** If you are receiving dialysis, your nutritional

requirements may change. Develop a specialized meal plan in close collaboration with a renal dietitian.

Foods to Limit or Avoid

It's important to limit or avoid certain foods that can be hard on the kidneys. Here's a list of foods to limit or avoid:

1. **High-Potassium Foods:** These can raise potassium levels in the blood, which can be harmful to the kidneys. Limit or avoid foods like bananas, oranges, potatoes, tomatoes, and spinach.

2. **High-Phosphorus Foods:** Too much phosphorus can be detrimental to kidney health. Limit or avoid foods like dairy products, nuts, seeds, and cola beverages.

3. **Sodium (Salt):** Excessive sodium intake can lead to high blood pressure and fluid retention, straining the kidneys. Avoid high-sodium foods like processed meats, canned soups, and fast food.

4. **Processed Foods:** These often contain high levels of sodium, phosphorus additives, and unhealthy fats. Limit or avoid packaged snacks, instant noodles, and processed meats.

5. **Red and Processed Meats:** These can be high in saturated fats and phosphorus. Limit your intake of red meats like beef and pork, and processed meats like sausages and bacon.

6. **Whole Grains:** While whole grains are generally healthy, they can be high in phosphorus. Choose white rice, pasta, and bread over whole grain options.

7. **Dairy Products:** Dairy products are high in phosphorus and potassium. Opt for

low-phosphorus alternatives like almond milk or limit your dairy intake.

8. **High-Sugar Foods:** Sugary foods and beverages can contribute to weight gain and high blood sugar levels, which can be problematic for kidney health. Limit sugary snacks, soda, and desserts.

9. **Caffeine:** Caffeine can raise blood pressure and cause dehydration. Limit coffee, tea, and caffeinated beverages.

10. **Alcohol:** Excessive alcohol consumption can affect kidney function and raise blood pressure. Drink alcohol in moderation or as advised by your healthcare provider.

11. **Certain Vegetables:** Some vegetables, like beets and Swiss chard, are high in oxalates, which can contribute to the formation of kidney stones. Limit these vegetables if you are prone to kidney stones.

12. **Avocado and Papaya:** While nutritious, these fruits are high in potassium and should be limited in a renal diet.

13. **Salt Substitutes:** Some salt substitutes contain high levels of potassium, which can be problematic. Consult with your healthcare provider before using them.

14. **Fatty Foods:** High-fat foods can contribute to weight gain and increase the risk of heart disease. Limit fried foods, butter, and fatty cuts of meat.

Cooking Techniques

1. **Portion Control:** One of the most important components of a renal diet is portion control. To prevent overfeeding the kidneys with extra nutrients, be cautious of portion amounts. To achieve precise portion amounts, use a kitchen scale and measuring cups.

2. **Limit Sodium:** Limit your salt intake because too much of it might cause fluid retention and elevated blood pressure. Use herbs and spices in place of salt to add flavor to your food while lowering the sodium content. Choose low- or no-sodium options when utilizing canned meals, and rinse the cans of veggies to get rid of the extra salt.

3. **Boiling and Steaming:** Instead of frying or sautéing your vegetables, think about boiling or steaming them. The demand for additional fats and salt is decreased while the nutrients are retained.

4. **Grilling and baking:** A fantastic approach to add flavor without adding a lot of salt or fat is to grill or bake proteins like chicken, fish, or lean meats. Use low-sodium marinades instead.

5. **Limit Phosphorus:** Limit your phosphorus intake because too much of it

can damage your kidneys. Reduce your intake of phosphorus-rich foods such dairy, almonds, and some beans. When feasible, choose low-phosphorus options.

6. **Dialysis-Friendly Proteins:** You might need to eat additional high-quality protein if you're on dialysis. Pick lean proteins such egg whites, fish, chicken, and turkey. To lower the phosphorus levels, remove the skin from the fowl.

7. **Use Fresh Ingredients:** Compared to canned or processed foods, fresh fruits and vegetables often have less salt and phosphorus. When it is available, include fresh produce in your meals.

8. **Limit Potassium:** Limit potassium intake by selecting fruits and vegetables with lower potassium content, such as apples, berries, and green beans, if your blood potassium levels are high. To remove some of the potassium before

cooking, soak foods high in potassium, such as potatoes.

9. **Homemade Stocks and Broths:** To reduce sodium intake when creating soups or stews, think about producing your own stocks and broths. Instead of salt, you can substitute herbs and spices for taste.

10. **Verify Labels:** Always read the salt, potassium, and phosphorus content on food labels. When purchasing, look for items expressly marked as "kidney-friendly."

11. **Keep Hydrated:** Kidney health depends on staying properly hydrated. Drink water all day long, but speak with your doctor about the best way to handle fluid consumption.

1. **Plan Your Meals:** Start by organizing your meals for the upcoming week. This will assist you in making a shopping list specifically for your renal diet, ensuring that you get the proper goods.

2. **Know the Dietary limits:** Become familiar with the dietary limits related to kidney health. These often include dietary restrictions for potassium, phosphorus, and sodium.

3. **Nutritional label reading:** Always pay close attention to food labels. Search for items with low-sodium, low-phosphorus, and low-potassium labels. To make informed decisions, be aware of serving sizes.

4. **Give Fresh Produce Priority:** A renal diet must include plenty of fresh fruits and vegetables. Choose low-potassium

foods such as green beans, cabbage, apples, and pears. Steer clear of foods high in potassium, such as oranges, potatoes, and spinach.

5. **Choose lean proteins:** Protein is important, but consuming too much might strain the kidneys. Pick skinless poultry, fish, and lean meat cuts as your lean protein sources. Look into vegetarian and vegan options as well, such as tofu, beans, and lentils.

6. **Be Wary of Processed Meats:** Meats that have been processed, such as bacon, sausages, and deli meats, frequently have high salt and phosphorus content. Choose low-sodium variants or consume these in moderation.

7. **Embrace Whole Grains:** Choose whole grains over refined grains, such as quinoa, brown rice, and whole wheat pasta. Because they include more dietary

fiber and less phosphorus, whole grains
are better for kidney function.

8. **Consider Your Dairy Options:** Dairy
products may include high levels of
potassium and phosphorus. Pick low-
phosphorus and low-potassium foods
such as small portions of plain Greek
yogurt, almond milk, or rice milk.

9. **Limit Your Sodium Intake:** Too much
sodium can cause fluid retention and
high blood pressure, both of which are
bad for your kidneys. Avoid adding extra
salt to your meals and use low-sodium or
salt-free goods.

10. **Season with Herbs and Spices:**
Use herbs and spices as a seasoning
alternative to salt to enhance the flavor
of your food. Your foods can taste
delicious when you add garlic powder,
basil, oregano, or rosemary.

11. **Avoid Sugary and Carbonated Beverages:** Avoid drinking sugary or fizzy beverages because they can cause weight gain and blood sugar swings. To stay hydrated, choose water, herbal tea, or unsweetened beverages.

12. **Consider Frozen or Canned Alternatives:** When fresh food is out of your price range or not easily accessible, think about frozen or canned fruits and vegetables without salt as viable alternatives.

CHAPTER 2:

BREAKFAST RECIPES

Greek Yogurt Parfait

Ingredients:

- 1 cup plain Greek yogurt

- 1/2 cup mixed berries (strawberries, blueberries, raspberries)

- 2 tablespoons chopped nuts (almonds, walnuts)

- 1 tablespoon honey (optional)

- Cinnamon for garnish (optional)

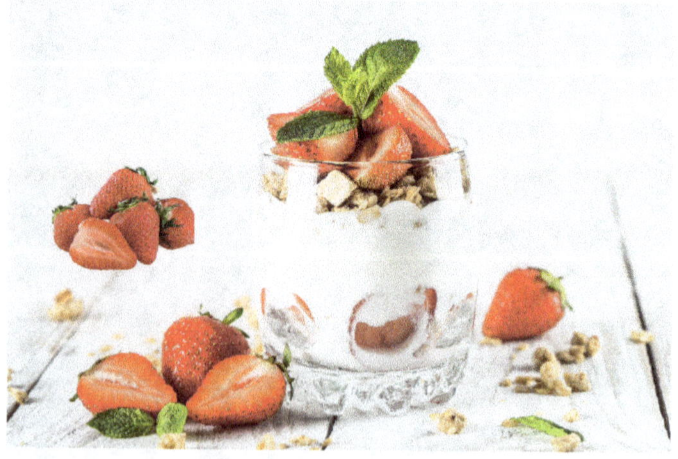

Nutritional Information:

Calories	Protein	Carbohydrates	Fat
250	20g	25g	9g

Preparation:

1. In a glass or bowl, layer the Greek yogurt, mixed berries, and chopped nuts.

2. Drizzle honey over the top if desired.

3. Sprinkle with a dash of cinnamon for added flavor.

4. Serve immediately.

Berry Smoothie

Ingredients:

- 1 cup mixed berries (strawberries, blueberries, raspberries)
- 1/2 ripe banana
- 1 cup unsweetened almond milk or low-potassium milk alternative

* 2 tablespoons Greek yogurt (optional for added creaminess)
* 1 tablespoon honey (optional)

Nutritional Information:

Calories	Protein	Carbohydrates	Fat
180	5g	40g	2g

Preparation:

1. Blend the mixed berries, banana, almond milk, and Greek yogurt until smooth.
2. Add honey for sweetness, if desired.
3. Pour into a glass and serve chilled.

Quinoa Breakfast Bowl

Ingredients:

* 1/2 cup cooked quinoa
* 1/4 cup sliced almonds
* 1/2 cup diced fresh fruit (such as apples or berries)

- 1 tablespoon honey or maple syrup (optional)
- Cinnamon for garnish (optional)

Nutritional Information:

Calories	Protein	Carbohydrates	Fat
300	10g	40g	8g

Preparation:

1. In a bowl, layer the cooked quinoa, sliced almonds, and diced fruit.
2. Drizzle honey or maple syrup for sweetness if desired.
3. Sprinkle with cinnamon.
4. Serve warm.

Oatmeal With Blueberries And Almonds

Ingredients:

- 1/2 cup rolled oats
- 1 cup water or low-potassium milk alternative
- 1/4 cup fresh blueberries
- 1 tablespoon chopped almonds
- 1 tablespoon honey or maple syrup (optional)

Nutritional Information:

Calories	Protein	Carbohydrates	Fat
250	7g	40g	6g

Preparation:

1. Cook the rolled oats with water or milk according to package instructions.
2. Top with fresh blueberries and chopped almonds.

3. Add honey or maple syrup for sweetness,
    if desired.

4. Serve hot.

Cottage Cheese and Peaches

Ingredients:

- 1/2 cup low-sodium cottage cheese
- 1 fresh peach (sliced)
- 1 tablespoon chopped pecans (optional)

Nutritional Information:

Calories	Protein	Carbohydrates	Fat
200	15g	20g	8g

Preparation:

1. Place cottage cheese in a bowl.

2. Top with sliced fresh peaches.

3. Sprinkle with chopped pecans, if desired.

4. Serve chilled.

Rice Cake with Peanut Butter

Ingredients:

- 1 rice cake (low-sodium)
- 2 tablespoons natural peanut butter (low-sodium)

Nutritional Information:

Calories	Protein	Carbohydrates	Fat
150	6g	15g	8g

Preparation:

1. Spread the peanut butter over the rice cake.
2. Serve as a healthy snack or quick breakfast option.

Vegetable And Mushroom Omelette

Ingredients:

- 2 eggs
- 1/4 cup diced bell peppers

- 1/4 cup sliced mushrooms

- 2 tablespoons chopped spinach

- 1 tablespoon olive oil

- Salt and pepper to taste

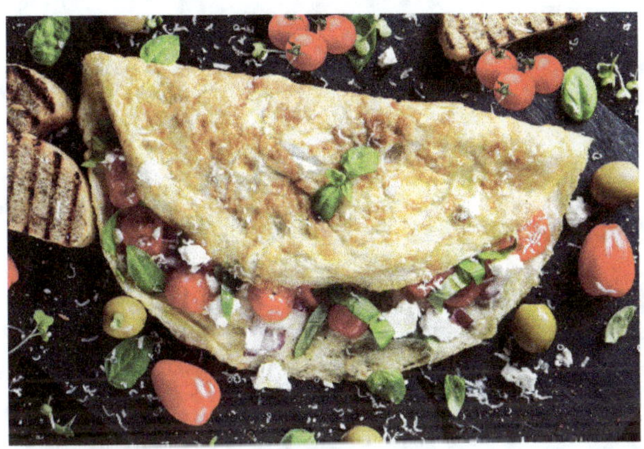

Nutritional Information:

Calories	Protein	Carbohydrates	Fat
250	15g	15g	18g

Preparation:

1. In a skillet, sauté the bell peppers, mushrooms, and spinach in olive oil until tender.

2. Whisk eggs and pour over the sautéed vegetables in the skillet.

3. Cook until the eggs are set and fold the omelette in half.

4. Season with salt and pepper.

5. Serve hot.

Homemade Low-Sodium Soup

Ingredients:

- 4 cups low-sodium vegetable or chicken broth
- 1 cup diced mixed vegetables (carrots, celery, onions)
- 1/2 cup diced potatoes
- 1/2 cup cooked quinoa or brown rice
- Herbs and spices (such as thyme, rosemary, and bay leaf)
- Salt-free seasoning blend
- Fresh parsley for garnish

Nutritional Information:

Calories	Protein	Carbohydrates	Fat
120	3g	25g	1g

Preparation:

1. In a pot, bring the broth to a simmer.
2. Add the mixed vegetables, potatoes, quinoa or rice, and herbs/spices.
3. Cook until the vegetables are tender.
4. Season with a salt-free seasoning blend.
5. Garnish with fresh parsley before serving.

Baked Apple

Ingredients:

- 1 large apple
- 1 teaspoon cinnamon
- 1 tablespoon chopped nuts (optional)
- 1 tablespoon honey (optional)

Nutritional Information:

Calories	Protein	Carbohydrates	Fat
100	1g	25g	0.5g

Preparation:

1. Preheat the oven to 350°F (175°C).
2. Core the apple and place it in a baking dish.
3. Sprinkle cinnamon over the apple.
4. Optionally, fill the core with chopped nuts and drizzle honey over the top.
5. Bake for 20-25 minutes or until the apple is tender.
6. Serve warm.

Almond Flour Pancakes with Blueberries

Ingredients:

- 1 cup almond flour
- 2 eggs

- 1/4 cup unsweetened almond milk or low-potassium milk alternative
- 1/2 teaspoon baking powder
- 1/2 cup fresh blueberries

Nutritional Information:

Calories	Protein	Carbohydrates	Fat
250	10g	10g	20g

Preparation:

1. In a bowl, mix almond flour, eggs, almond milk, and baking powder until well combined.
2. Gently fold in the fresh blueberries.
3. Heat a non-stick skillet over medium heat and pour batter to make pancakes.
4. Cook until bubbles form, then flip and cook the other side.
5. Serve with fresh fruit or sugar-free syrup.

Rice Pudding

Ingredients:

- 1/2 cup cooked white rice
- 1 cup low-potassium milk alternative
- 1 tablespoon honey or maple syrup (optional)
- 1/2 teaspoon vanilla extract
- Ground cinnamon for garnish (optional)

Nutritional Information:

Calories	Protein	Carbohydrates	Fat
200	4g	40g	3g

Preparation:

1. In a saucepan, combine the cooked rice and low-potassium milk.
2. Bring to a simmer over medium heat, stirring frequently.
3. Stir in honey or maple syrup and vanilla extract.

4. Cook until the mixture thickens to a creamy consistency.

5. Sprinkle it with ground cinnamon and serve warm.

Egg and Vegetable Breakfast Burrito

Ingredients:

- 2 eggs
- 1/4 cup diced bell peppers
- 1/4 cup chopped spinach
- 2 low-sodium whole grain tortillas
- Salsa or low-sodium hot sauce (optional)

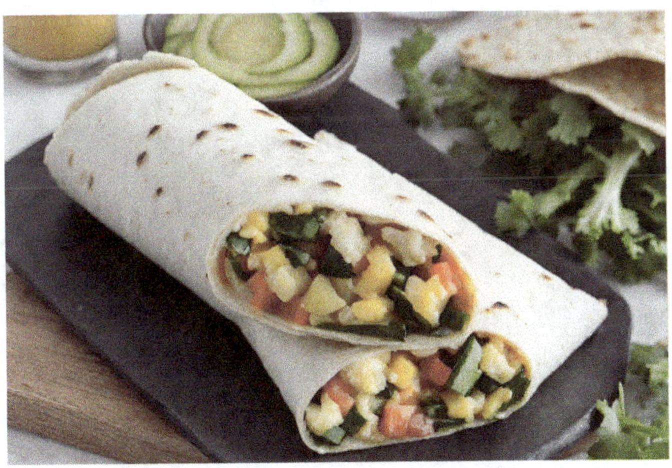

Nutritional Information:

Calories	Protein	Carbohydrates	Fat
300	15g	30g	12g

Preparation:

1. In a skillet, scramble the eggs with diced bell peppers and chopped spinach.
2. Warm the tortillas in the skillet or microwave.
3. Place the egg and vegetable mixture onto the tortillas.
4. Roll up the tortillas, tucking in the sides to form a burrito.
5. Serve with salsa or low-sodium hot sauce if desired.

Low-Potassium Smoothie

Ingredients:

- 1/2 ripe banana
- 1/2 cup unsweetened applesauce

- 1/2 cup fresh spinach

- 1/2 cup low-potassium milk alternative

- 1 tablespoon almond butter (optional)

Nutritional Information:

Calories	Protein	Carbohydrates	Fat
200	5g	35g	5g

Preparation:

1. Blend the banana, applesauce, spinach, and low-potassium milk until smooth.

2. Add almond butter for extra creaminess if desired.

3. Pour into a glass and serve chilled.

Buckwheat Pancakes

Ingredients:

- 1 cup buckwheat flour

- 1 tablespoon honey or maple syrup

- 1 egg

- 1 cup low-potassium milk alternative
- 1/2 teaspoon baking powder
- Fresh fruit for topping (optional)

Nutritional Information:

Calories	Protein	Carbohydrates	Fat
250	8g	40g	5g

Preparation:

1. In a bowl, mix buckwheat flour, honey or maple syrup, egg, milk, and baking powder until well combined.
2. Heat a non-stick skillet over medium heat and pour batter to make pancakes.
3. Cook until bubbles form, then flip and cook the other side.
4. Serve with fresh fruit if desired.

Homemade Muesli

Ingredients:

- 1 cup rolled oats
- 1/4 cup chopped nuts (almonds, walnuts)
- 1/4 cup dried fruit (raisins, cranberries)
- 1 tablespoon chia seeds
- Cinnamon for flavor (optional)

Nutritional Information:

Calories	Protein	Carbohydrates	Fat
200	6g	30g	7g

Preparation:

1. Mix all the ingredients in a bowl.
2. Store in an airtight container for a ready-to-eat breakfast option.
3. Serve with low-potassium milk alternative or yogurt.

Cinnamon Raisin Toast

Ingredients:

- 2 slices low-sodium whole grain bread
- 1 tablespoon unsalted butter or margarine (optional)
- 1 teaspoon ground cinnamon
- 2 tablespoons raisins

Nutritional Information:

Calories	Protein	Carbohydrates	Fat
200	5g	35g	5g

Preparation:

1. Toast the whole grain bread slices.
2. Spread unsalted butter or margarine if using.
3. Sprinkle ground cinnamon over the toast.
4. Top with raisins and serve.

Low-Sodium Breakfast Casserole

Ingredients:

- 4 eggs

- 1 cup low-fat shredded cheese

- 1 cup diced vegetables (bell peppers, onions, spinach)

- 1/2 cup low-sodium ham or turkey, diced

- Salt-free seasoning blend

- Fresh parsley for garnish

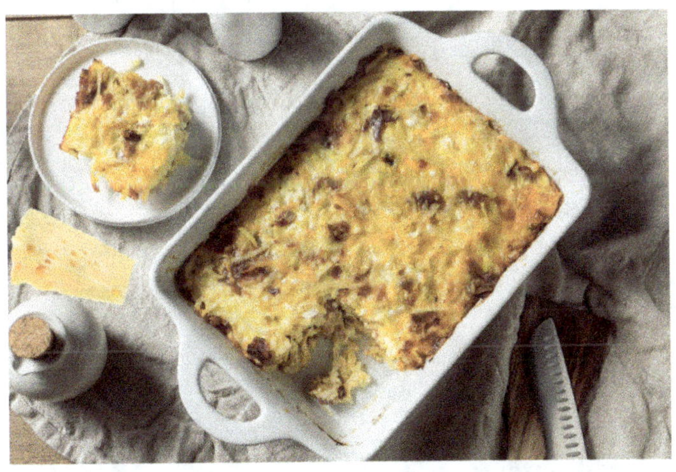

Nutritional Information:

Calories	Protein	Carbohydrates	Fat
200	15g	5g	10g

Preparation:

1. Preheat oven to 350°F (175°C).

2. In a bowl, whisk the eggs and salt-free seasoning blend.

3. Stir in the cheese, diced vegetables, and diced ham or turkey.

4. Pour the mixture into a greased baking dish.

5. Bake for 25-30 minutes until set and slightly golden.

6. Garnish with fresh parsley before serving.

Chia Pudding With Berries

Ingredients:

- 3 tablespoons chia seeds
- 1 cup low-potassium milk alternative
- 1/2 cup mixed berries

- 1 tablespoon honey or maple syrup (optional)

Nutritional Information:

Calories	Protein	Carbohydrates	Fat
180	5g	25g	7g

Preparation:

1. In a bowl, mix chia seeds and low-potassium milk.
2. Refrigerate for at least 2 hours or overnight to allow the chia seeds to expand and form a pudding-like consistency.
3. Top with mixed berries and drizzle with honey or maple syrup if desired.
4. Serve chilled.

CHAPTER 3:

LUNCH IDEAS

Grilled Chicken Salad with Mixed Greens

Ingredients:

- 4 oz grilled chicken breast, sliced
- Mixed salad greens (spinach, arugula, lettuce)
- Sliced cucumbers and cherry tomatoes
- 2 tablespoons balsamic vinaigrette (low-sodium)

Nutritional Information:

Calories	Protein	Carbohydrates	Fat
250	25g	10g	12g

Preparation:

1. Arrange mixed greens, cucumbers, and cherry tomatoes on a plate.

2. Top with grilled chicken slices.

3. Drizzle with balsamic vinaigrette and serve.

Baked Salmon with Lemon and Dill

Ingredients:

- 6 oz salmon fillet
- Slices of lemon
- Fresh dill
- Salt and pepper to taste

Nutritional Information:

Calories	Protein	Carbohydrates	Fat
300	30g	0g	18g

Preparation:

1. Preheat the oven to 375°F (190°C).
2. Place the salmon on a baking sheet.
3. Season with salt, pepper, and fresh dill.
4. Top with slices of lemon.
5. Bake for 15-20 minutes or until the salmon is cooked through.
6. Serve hot.

Tuna Salad with Low-Sodium Dressing

Ingredients:

- 5 oz canned tuna (in water, drained)
- Chopped celery and red onions
- Low-sodium mayonnaise
- Dijon mustard
- Salt-free seasoning blend

Nutritional Information:

Calories	Protein	Carbohydrates	Fat
200	20g	5g	10g

Preparation:

1. In a bowl, mix the drained tuna, chopped celery, and red onions.

2. Add low-sodium mayonnaise, Dijon mustard, and seasoning blend to taste.

3. Stir until well combined and serve as a salad or in a sandwich.

Quinoa and Vegetable Stir-Fry

Ingredients:

- 1 cup cooked quinoa
- Assorted vegetables (bell peppers, broccoli, carrots, snap peas)
- Low-sodium soy sauce
- Minced garlic and ginger
- Olive oil

Nutritional Information:

Calories	Protein	Carbohydrates	Fat

250	8g	40g	6g

Preparation:

1. Heat olive oil in a pan or wok.

2. Sauté minced garlic and ginger.

3. Add assorted vegetables and stir-fry until tender-crisp.

4. Stir in cooked quinoa and a splash of low-sodium soy sauce.

5. Cook for a few more minutes and serve hot.

Turkey and Avocado Wrap with Whole-Grain Tortilla

Ingredients:

- 4 oz sliced turkey breast
- 1/4 ripe avocado, sliced
- Shredded lettuce and sliced tomatoes
- Whole-grain tortilla
- Low-sodium mayonnaise (optional)

Nutritional Information:

Calories	Protein	Carbohydrates	Fat
300	25g	25g	10g

Preparation:

1. Lay out the tortilla and spread low-sodium mayonnaise if desired.

2. Layer with sliced turkey, avocado, shredded lettuce, and sliced tomatoes.

3. Roll up the tortilla, slice in half, and serve.

Vegetable and Chicken Kebabs

Ingredients:

- 4 oz chicken breast, cubed
- Assorted vegetables (bell peppers, onions, zucchini)
- Olive oil
- Herbs and spices of choice

- Skewers

Nutritional Information:

Calories	Protein	Carbohydrates	Fat
200	20g	10g	8g

Preparation:

1. Preheat grill to medium-high heat.

2. Thread chicken and assorted vegetables onto skewers.

3. Brush with olive oil and season with herbs and spices.

4. Grill for 10-15 minutes, turning occasionally until chicken is cooked through and vegetables are tender.

Lentil and Vegetable Curry

Ingredients:

- 1 cup cooked lentils
- Assorted vegetables (eggplant, cauliflower, bell peppers)
- Curry powder
- Coconut milk (low-fat)
- Chopped cilantro for garnish

Nutritional Information:

Calories	Protein	Carbohydrates	Fat
300	15g	40g	8g

Preparation:

1. Sauté assorted vegetables in a pan.
2. Add cooked lentils, curry powder, and coconut milk.
3. Simmer for 10-15 minutes until vegetables are tender and the curry thickens.

4. Garnish with chopped cilantro and serve
    with rice or quinoa.

Grilled Shrimp with Lemon Garlic Sauce

Ingredients:

- 6 oz shrimp, peeled and deveined
- Minced garlic
- Lemon juice
- Olive oil
- Chopped parsley for garnish

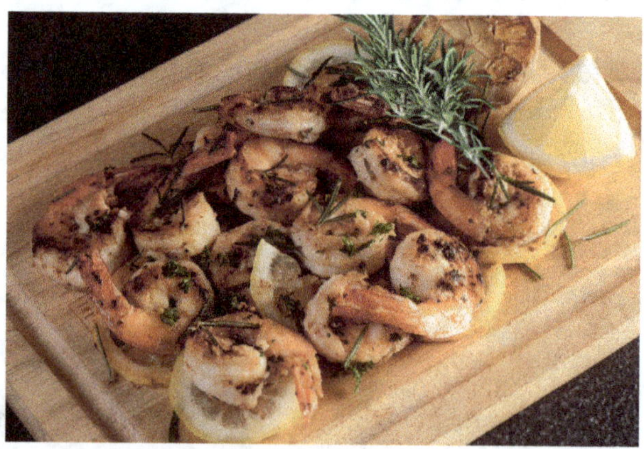

Nutritional Information:

Calories	Protein	Carbohydrates	Fat
200	25g	2g	10g

Preparation:

1. In a bowl, mix shrimp with minced garlic, lemon juice, and a drizzle of olive oil.

2. Marinate for 15-30 minutes.

3. Grill shrimp over medium heat for 2-3 minutes per side until cooked.

4. Garnish with chopped parsley and serve.

Turkey and Vegetable Stir-Fry

Ingredients:

- 4 oz sliced turkey
- Assorted vegetables (snow peas, carrots, bell peppers)
- Low-sodium stir-fry sauce
- Sesame oil
- Cooked brown rice

Nutritional Information:

Calories	Protein	Carbohydrates	Fat
250	20g	30g	6g

Preparation:

1. Heat sesame oil in a pan or wok.

2. Stir-fry turkey slices until cooked through.

3. Add assorted vegetables and stir-fry until tender.

4. Stir in low-sodium stir-fry sauce and serve over cooked brown rice.

Roasted Red Pepper and Chickpea Salad

Ingredients:

- Roasted red peppers, sliced
- Cooked chickpeas
- Chopped parsley
- Olive oil and balsamic vinegar

- Crumbled feta cheese (optional)

Nutritional Information:

Calories	Protein	Carbohydrates	Fat
220	8g	25g	10g

Preparation:

1. Combine roasted red peppers and cooked chickpeas in a bowl.
2. Drizzle with olive oil and balsamic vinegar.
3. Sprinkle chopped parsley and crumbled feta cheese if desired.
4. Toss to combine and serve.

Grilled Pork Tenderloin with Herbs

Ingredients:

- 6 oz pork tenderloin
- Herbs (rosemary, thyme)
- Garlic powder

- Olive oil

Nutritional Information:

Calories	Protein	Carbohydrates	Fat
250	30g	0g	12g

Preparation:

1. Preheat the grill to medium-high heat.
2. Rub pork tenderloin with herbs, garlic powder, and a touch of olive oil.
3. Grill for about 15-20 minutes, turning occasionally until internal temperature reaches 145°F (63°C).
4. Let it rest for a few minutes before slicing and serving.

Chicken and Rice Soup

Ingredients:

- Cooked chicken breast, shredded
- Cooked brown rice

- Chopped carrots, celery, and onions

- Low-sodium chicken broth

- Herbs (thyme, parsley)

- Salt and pepper to taste

Nutritional Information:

Calories	Protein	Carbohydrates	Fat
200	15g	20g	5g

Preparation:

1. In a pot, combine chopped vegetables, chicken broth, and herbs.

2. Simmer until vegetables are tender.

3. Add cooked chicken and rice.

4. Season with salt and pepper to taste and serve hot.

Roasted Vegetable and Feta Quiche

Ingredients:

- Pie crust (store-bought or homemade)
- Assorted roasted vegetables (zucchini, bell peppers, onions)
- Crumbled feta cheese
- 4 eggs
- Low-fat milk or low-potassium milk alternative

Nutritional Information:

Calories	Protein	Carbohydrates	Fat
250	10g	20g	15g

Preparation:

1. Preheat oven to 375°F (190°C).
2. Place the pie crust in a pie dish.
3. Layer roasted vegetables and crumbled feta cheese in the pie crust.
4. In a bowl, whisk together eggs and milk.

5. Pour the egg mixture over the vegetables and cheese.

6. Bake for 30-35 minutes or until the quiche is set and slightly golden on top.

Tofu and Vegetable Teriyaki Stir-Fry

Ingredients:

- Firm tofu, cubed
- Assorted vegetables (broccoli, bell peppers, snow peas)
- Low-sodium teriyaki sauce
- Sesame oil
- Cooked brown rice

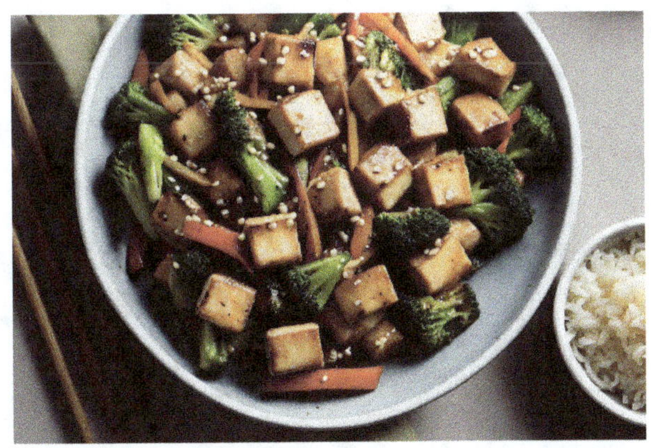

Nutritional Information:

Calories	Protein	Carbohydrates	Fat
300	15g	35g	10g

Preparation:

1. Heat sesame oil in a pan or wok.

2. Stir-fry tofu until lightly browned.

3. Add assorted vegetables and stir-fry until tender.

4. Stir in low-sodium teriyaki sauce and serve over cooked brown rice.

Greek Salad with Low-Potassium Olives

Ingredients:

- Mixed salad greens
- Sliced cucumbers and cherry tomatoes
- Low-potassium olives
- Crumbled feta cheese
- Olive oil and red wine vinegar

Nutritional Information:

Calories	Protein	Carbohydrates	Fat
200	5g	10g	15g

Preparation:

1. Combine mixed greens, cucumbers, and cherry tomatoes in a bowl.

2. Add low-potassium olives and crumbled feta cheese.

3. Drizzle with olive oil and red wine vinegar, toss, and serve.

Roast Beef and Swiss Cheese Sandwich on Whole-Grain Bread

Ingredients:

- Thinly sliced roast beef
- Swiss cheese slices
- Lettuce and sliced tomatoes
- Whole-grain bread
- Dijon mustard (optional)

Nutritional Information:

Calories	Protein	Carbohydrates	Fat
300	25g	25g	10g

Preparation:

1. Layer roast beef, Swiss cheese, lettuce, and tomatoes on whole-grain bread.
2. Spread Dijon mustard if desired.
3. Serve as a satisfying sandwich option.

Ratatouille with Herbs

Ingredients:

- Assorted vegetables (eggplant, zucchini, bell peppers)
- Diced tomatoes
- Minced garlic and onion
- Herbs (thyme, rosemary, basil)

Nutritional Information:

Calories	Protein	Carbohydrates	Fat
150	5g	20g	5g

Preparation:

1. Sauté minced garlic and onion in a pan.

2. Add assorted vegetables and diced tomatoes.

3. Season with herbs and simmer until vegetables are tender.

4. Serve as a side dish or over whole-grain pasta.

Turkey Chili with Kidney-Friendly Beans

Ingredients:

- Ground turkey
- Kidney beans (low-sodium, if canned)
- Chopped tomatoes
- Diced bell peppers and onions

- Chili powder and cumin

Nutritional Information:

Calories	Protein	Carbohydrates	Fat
250	20g	20g	10g

Preparation:

1. Brown ground turkey in a pot.

2. Add chopped tomatoes, diced vegetables, kidney beans, and spices.

3. Simmer for 20-30 minutes until flavors meld together.

4. Serve as a hearty and flavorful chili.

Spinach and Feta Stuffed Chicken Breast

Ingredients:

- Boneless, skinless chicken breasts
- Fresh spinach leaves
- Crumbled feta cheese

- Minced garlic
- Olive oil

Nutritional Information:

Calories	Protein	Carbohydrates	Fat
300	30g	5g	15g

Preparation:

1. Preheat the oven to 375°F (190°C).
2. Cut a pocket into the side of each chicken breast.
3. Stuff with fresh spinach and crumbled feta cheese.
4. Rub the chicken with minced garlic and a touch of olive oil.
5. Bake for 25-30 minutes or until the chicken is fully cooked.

CHAPTER 4:

DINNER DELIGHTS

Baked Lemon Herb Chicken

Ingredients:

- 4 boneless, skinless chicken breasts
- Lemon juice
- Chopped fresh herbs (such as thyme, rosemary, and parsley)
- Garlic powder
- Olive oil

Nutritional Information:

Calories	Protein	Carbohydrates	Fat
200	25g	0g	10g

Preparation:

1. Preheat the oven to 375°F (190°C).

2. Place the chicken breasts in a baking dish.

3. Drizzle with lemon juice and olive oil.

4. Sprinkle chopped herbs and garlic powder over the chicken.

5. Bake for 25-30 minutes or until the chicken reaches an internal temperature of 165°F (74°C).

Grilled Salmon with Dill Sauce

Ingredients:

- 4 salmon fillets
- Lemon juice
- Chopped fresh dill
- Salt and pepper
- Low-fat sour cream (or low-potassium yogurt)

Nutritional Information:

Calories	Protein	Carbohydrates	Fat
250	25g	2g	15g

Preparation:

1. Preheat the grill to medium-high heat.

2. Season salmon fillets with salt, pepper, and lemon juice.

3. Grill for 4-5 minutes per side until the fish flakes easily with a fork.

4. Mix chopped dill with low-fat sour cream or low-potassium yogurt for a sauce to serve alongside the grilled salmon.

Vegetable Stir-Fry

Ingredients:

- Assorted vegetables (bell peppers, broccoli, carrots, snap peas)
- Low-sodium stir-fry sauce

- Sesame oil

- Cooked brown rice or quinoa

Nutritional Information:

Calories	Protein	Carbohydrates	Fat
150	5g	20g	5g

Preparation:

1. Heat sesame oil in a pan or wok.

2. Stir-fry assorted vegetables until tender-crisp.

3. Add low-sodium stir-fry sauce and cook for a few more minutes.

4. Serve over cooked brown rice or quinoa.

Turkey and Vegetable Soup

Ingredients:

- Cooked turkey (shredded)

- Diced vegetables (carrots, celery, onions)

- Low-sodium chicken or vegetable broth

- Herbs (thyme, parsley)
- Salt and pepper to taste

Nutritional Information:

Calories	Protein	Carbohydrates	Fat
200	15g	15g	8g

Preparation:

1. In a pot, combine diced vegetables, cooked turkey, and broth.and
2. Simmer until the vegetables are tender.
3. Season with herbs, salt, pepper to taste.
4. Serve the soup hot.

Baked Cod with Tomato and Basil

Ingredients:

- Cod fillets
- Chopped tomatoes
- Chopped fresh basil
- Minced garlic

- Olive oil

Nutritional Information:

Calories	Protein	Carbohydrates	Fat
150	20g	5g	5g

Preparation:

1. Preheat the oven to 375°F (190°C).

2. Place the cod fillets in a baking dish.

3. Top with chopped tomatoes, minced garlic, and fresh basil.

4. Drizzle with olive oil.

5. Bake for 15-20 minutes or until the fish is cooked through.

Spinach and Mushroom Stuffed Chicken

Ingredients:

- Boneless, skinless chicken breasts

- Fresh spinach leaves

- Sliced mushrooms

- Minced garlic

- Low-fat mozzarella cheese

Nutritional Information:

Calories	Protein	Carbohydrates	Fat
250	30g	5g	10g

Preparation:

1. Preheat the oven to 375°F (190°C).

2. Cut a pocket into the side of each chicken breast.

3. Stuff with fresh spinach, sliced mushrooms, minced garlic, and a sprinkle of low-fat mozzarella cheese.

4. Bake for 25-30 minutes or until the chicken is fully cooked.

Lemon Garlic Shrimp

Ingredients:

- Shrimp, peeled and deveined
- Minced garlicLemon juice
- Olive oil
- Chopped parsley for garnish

Nutritional Information:

Calories	Protein	Carbohydrates	Fat
150	20g	2g	7g

Preparation:

1. Heat olive oil in a pan.
2. Sauté minced garlic until fragrant.
3. Add shrimp and cook for 2-3 minutes per side until pink and cooked through.
4. Squeeze fresh lemon juice over the shrimp and garnish with chopped parsley before serving.

Quinoa and Black Bean Salad

Ingredients:

- Cooked quinoa
- Black beans (rinsed and drained)
- Diced bell peppers and red onions
- Chopped cilantro
- Lime juice and olive oil

Nutritional Information:

Calories	Protein	Carbohydrates	Fat
200	8g	30g	6g

Preparation:

1. In a bowl, mix cooked quinoa, black beans, diced bell peppers, red onions, and chopped cilantro.
2. Drizzle with lime juice and olive oil.
3. Toss to combine and serve as a refreshing salad.

Eggplant Parmesan

Ingredients:

- Sliced eggplant
- Breadcrumbs (or almond flour for a lower carb option)
- Egg or egg substitute
- Marinara sauce (low-sodium)
- Shredded mozzarella cheese (low-fat)

Nutritional Information:

Calories	Protein	Carbohydrates	Fat
250	10g	20g	12g

Preparation:

1. Preheat the oven to 375°F (190°C).
2. Dip eggplant slices in egg, then coat with breadcrumbs or almond flour.
3. Place on a baking sheet and bake for 20-25 minutes until golden.

4. In a baking dish, layer marinara sauce, baked eggplant, and shredded mozzarella cheese.

5. Bake for an additional 15-20 minutes until the cheese is melted and bubbly.

Turkey and Vegetable Skewers

Ingredients:

- Cubed turkey breast
- Assorted vegetables (bell peppers, onions, zucchini)
- Olive oil
- Herbs and spices of choice

Nutritional Information:

Calories	Protein	Carbohydrates	Fat
200	20g	10g	8g

Preparation:

1. Preheat the grill to medium-high heat.

2. Thread turkey cubes and assorted vegetables onto skewers.

3. Brush with olive oil and season with herbs and spices.

4. Grill for 10-15 minutes, turning occasionally until turkey is cooked through and vegetables are tender.

Grilled Portobello Mushrooms

Ingredients:

- Portobello mushroom caps
- Balsamic vinegar
- Minced garlic
- Olive oil

Nutritional Information:

Calories	Protein	Carbohydrates	Fat
50	3g	5g	3g

Preparation:

1. Mix balsamic vinegar, minced garlic, and olive oil in a bowl.
2. Marinate mushroom caps in the mixture for 15-30 minutes.
3. Preheat the grill to medium heat.
4. Grill mushrooms for 4-5 minutes on each side until tender.

Lemon Herb Roasted Chicken Thighs

Ingredients:

- Chicken thighs, bone-in and skin-on
- Lemon zest and juice
- Chopped fresh herbs (thyme, oregano, parsley)
- Minced garlic
- Olive oil

Nutritional Information:

Calories	Protein	Carbohydrates	Fat

250	20g	0g		18g

Preparation:

1. Preheat the oven to 400°F (200°C).

2. Mix lemon zest, lemon juice, chopped herbs, minced garlic, and olive oil in a bowl.

3. Rub the mixture over the chicken thighs.

4. Place the chicken on a baking sheet and roast for 35-40 minutes or until cooked through.

Tofu and Vegetable Stir-Fry

Ingredients:

- Firm tofu, cubed
- Assorted vegetables (broccoli, bell peppers, snow peas)
- Low-sodium stir-fry sauce
- Sesame oil
- Cooked brown rice

Nutritional Information:

Calories	Protein	Carbohydrates	Fat
250	15g	30g	8g

Preparation:

1. Heat sesame oil in a pan or wok.

2. Stir-fry tofu until lightly browned.

3. Add assorted vegetables and stir-fry until tender.

4. Stir in low-sodium stir-fry sauce and serve over cooked brown rice.

Baked Zucchini and Tomato Casserole

Ingredients:

- Sliced zucchini and tomatoes
- Minced garlic
- Olive oil
- Herbs (thyme, basil)
- Parmesan cheese (low-sodium)

Nutritional Information:

Calories	Protein	Carbohydrates	Fat
150	5g	10g	10g

Preparation:

1. Preheat the oven to 375°F (190°C).

2. Arrange alternating slices of zucchini and tomato in a baking dish.

3. Drizzle with olive oil, minced garlic, and sprinkle with herbs.

4. Bake for 20-25 minutes, then top with low-sodium Parmesan cheese and bake for an additional 5-10 minutes.

Baked Pork Chops with Apples

Ingredients:

- Pork chops
- Sliced apples
- Cinnamon

- Brown sugar substitute (for lower sugar option)
- Olive oil

Nutritional Information:

Calories	Protein	Carbohydrates	Fat
250	30g	10g	10g

Preparation:

1. Preheat the oven to 375°F (190°C).
2. Season pork chops with cinnamon and a sprinkle of brown sugar substitute.
3. Top with sliced apples and drizzle with a touch of olive oil.
4. Bake for 20-25 minutes or until pork is cooked through.

Roasted Butternut Squash Soup

Ingredients:

- Peeled and cubed butternut squash
- Chopped onions and carrots
- Low-sodium vegetable or chicken broth
- Herbs (thyme, sage)
- Salt and pepper to taste

Nutritional Information:

Calories	Protein	Carbohydrates	Fat
150	2g	30g	1g

Preparation:

1. Roast cubed butternut squash, onions, and carrots until tender.
2. Blend the roasted vegetables with low-sodium broth until smooth.
3. Pour the mixture into a pot, add herbs, salt, and pepper.

4. Simmer for a few minutes and serve the soup hot.

Chicken and Asparagus Stir-Fry

Ingredients:

- Sliced chicken breast
- Asparagus spears, cut into pieces
- Low-sodium soy sauce
- Minced ginger and garlic
- Sesame oil

Nutritional Information:

Calories	Protein	Carbohydrates	Fat
200	20g	10g	8g

Preparation:

1. Heat sesame oil in a pan or wok.
2. Stir-fry sliced chicken until cooked through.

3. Add asparagus, minced ginger, and garlic, and continue to stir-fry until the asparagus is tender-crisp.

4. Drizzle with low-sodium soy sauce and serve hot.

Grilled Tofu with Pesto

Ingredients:

- Firm tofu slices
- Pesto sauce (low-sodium)
- Olive oil
- Herbs for garnish

Nutritional Information:

Calories	Protein	Carbohydrates	Fat
180	15g	10g	10g

Preparation:

1. Preheat the grill to medium-high heat.

2. Brush tofu slices with olive oil.

3. Grill for 3-4 minutes per side until grill marks appear.

4. Serve with a dollop of low-sodium pesto sauce and garnish with fresh herbs.

Baked Sweet Potato and Black Bean Enchiladas

Ingredients:

- Cooked and mashed sweet potatoes
- Black beans (low-sodium, drained)
- Whole-grain tortillas
- Enchilada sauce (low-sodium)
- Shredded low-fat cheese

Nutritional Information:

Calories	Protein	Carbohydrates	Fat
250	10g	30g	8g

Preparation

1. Preheat the oven to 375°F (190°C).

2. Mix mashed sweet potatoes and black beans.

3. Spoon the mixture onto tortillas, roll them up, and place in a baking dish.

4. Pour low-sodium enchilada sauce over the top, sprinkle with low-fat cheese, and bake for 20-25 minutes.

Baked Chicken with Roasted Vegetables

Ingredients:

- Chicken pieces (thighs, drumsticks)
- Assorted vegetables (bell peppers, onions, carrots)
- Olive oil
- Herbs and spices

Nutritional Information:

Calories	Protein	Carbohydrates	Fat
250	25g	10g	12g

Preparation:

1. Preheat the oven to 375°F (190°C).
2. Arrange chicken pieces and chopped vegetables in a baking dish.
3. Drizzle with olive oil, season with herbs and spices, and toss to coat.
4. Bake for 40-45 minutes or until the chicken is cooked through and vegetables are tender.

Chili Lime Shrimp Tacos

Ingredients:

- Shrimp, peeled and deveined
- Chili powder
- Lime juice
- Whole-grain tortillas
- Shredded cabbage and salsa for garnish

Nutritional Information:

Calories	Protein	Carbohydrates	Fat
250	20g	30g	5g

Preparation:

1. Season shrimp with chili powder and lime juice.

2. Sauté the seasoned shrimp in a pan until cooked.

3. Warm tortillas, fill with shrimp, shredded cabbage, and salsa.

Baked Eggplant and Tomato Stacks

Ingredients:

- Sliced eggplant and tomatoes
- Minced garlic
- Olive oil
- Herbs (basil, oregano)
- Low-fat mozzarella cheese

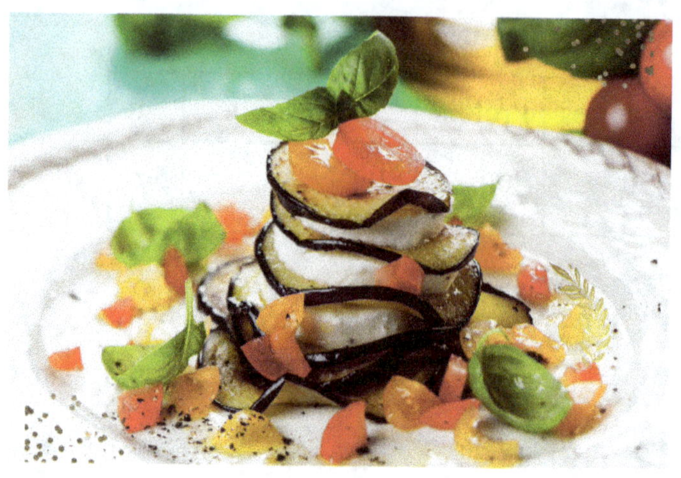

Nutritional Information:

Calories	Protein	Carbohydrates	Fat
100	5g	10g	5g

Preparation:

1. Preheat the oven to 375°F (190°C).

2. Layer alternating slices of eggplant and tomato on a baking sheet.

3. Drizzle with olive oil, sprinkle with minced garlic and herbs.

4. Top with low-fat mozzarella cheese and bake for 20-25 minutes.

Sesame Ginger Tofu and Broccoli

Ingredients:

- Firm tofu, cubed
- Broccoli florets
- Low-sodium soy sauce
- Minced ginger
- Sesame seeds

Nutritional Information:

Calories	Protein	Carbohydrates	Fat
180	15g	10g	8g

Preparation:

1. In a pan, stir-fry cubed tofu until lightly browned.
2. Add broccoli, minced ginger, and a splash of low-sodium soy sauce.
3. Cook until the broccoli is tender, sprinkle with sesame seeds, and serve.

Healthy Snacking

Cucumber and Cottage Cheese Snack

Ingredients:

- Cucumber, sliced
- Low-fat cottage cheese
- Dill or chives (for garnish, optional)

Nutritional Information:

Calories	Protein	Carbohydrates	Fat
80	8g	5g	3g

Preparation:

1. Place a dollop of low-fat cottage cheese on each cucumber slice.
2. Garnish with dill or chives if desired and enjoy this simple, low-calorie snack.

Apple and Almond Butter Slices

Ingredients:

- Apple, sliced
- Almond butter (low-sodium)

Nutritional Information:

Calories	Protein	Carbohydrates	Fat
120	3g	20g	5g

Preparation:

1. Spread almond butter on apple slices for a tasty and nutritious snack rich in fiber and healthy fats.

Greek Yogurt with Berries

Ingredients:

- Low-fat Greek yogurt
- Mixed berries (blueberries, strawberries, raspberries)

Nutritional Information:

Calories	Protein	Carbohydrates	Fat
100	10g	15g	2g

Preparation:

1. Top a portion of low-fat Greek yogurt with mixed berries for a protein-packed and antioxidant-rich snack.

Popcorn with Herbs

Ingredients:

- Unsalted popcorn
- Herbs (like rosemary, thyme, or nutritional yeast for flavor)

Nutritional Information:

Calories	Protein	Carbohydrates	Fat
50	1g	10g	1g

Preparation:

1. Air-pop unsalted popcorn and sprinkle with herbs or nutritional yeast for a flavorful, low-calorie snack.

Carrot Sticks with Hummus

Ingredients:

- Carrot sticks
- Low-sodium hummus

Nutritional Information:

Calories	Protein	Carbohydrates	Fat
70	3g	10g	3g

Preparation:

1. Dip carrot sticks in low-sodium hummus for a snack that's rich in fiber and plant-based protein.

Tuna Salad on Whole-Grain Crackers

Ingredients:

- Canned tuna (packed in water), drained
- Low-fat mayonnaise
- Diced celery and onion
- Whole-grain crackers

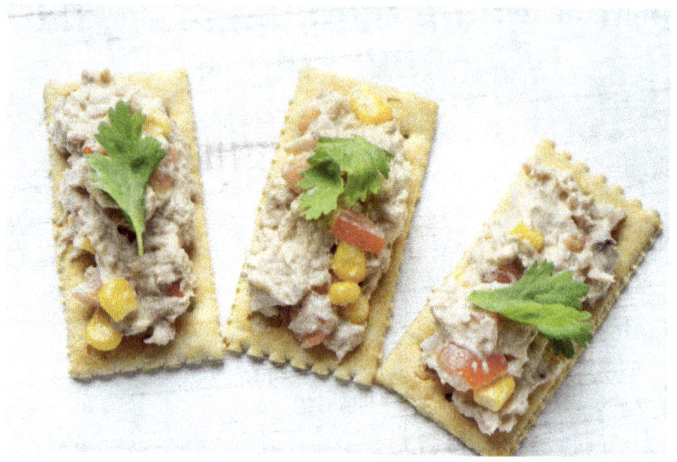

Nutritional Information:

Calories	Protein	Carbohydrates	Fat
150	15g	10g	5g

Preparation:

1. Mix drained tuna with low-fat mayonnaise, diced celery, and onion.
2. Spread on whole-grain crackers for a protein-rich and satisfying snack.

Rice Cake with Almond Butter and Banana Slices

Ingredients:

- Whole-grain rice cake
- Almond butter (low-sodium)
- Banana, sliced

Nutritional Information:

Calories	Protein	Carbohydrates	Fat
130	3g	20g	5g

Preparation:

1. Spread almond butter on a whole-grain rice cake and top with banana slices for a quick and energy-boosting snack.

Avocado Toast on Whole-Grain Bread

Ingredients:

- Mashed avocado
- Whole-grain bread, toasted
- Sliced tomatoes or a sprinkle of black pepper (optional)

Nutritional Information:

Calories	Protein	Carbohydrates	Fat
150	5g	20g	7g

Preparation:

1. Spread mashed avocado on toasted whole-grain bread for a nutrient-rich snack loaded with healthy fats.

Quinoa and Vegetable Salad

Ingredients:

- Cooked quinoa
- Diced cucumbers, bell peppers, and cherry tomatoes
- Chopped parsley
- Olive oil and lemon juice

Nutritional Information:

Calories	Protein	Carbohydrates	Fat
150	5g	20g	5g

Preparation:

1. Mix cooked quinoa with diced vegetables and chopped parsley.
2. Drizzle with olive oil and lemon juice for a refreshing and nutritious salad.

Steamed Asparagus with Lemon Zest

Ingredients:

- Fresh asparagus spears
- Lemon zest
- Olive oil
- Salt and pepper

Nutritional Information:

Calories	Protein	Carbohydrates	Fat
40	3g	5g	2g

Preparation:

1. Steam asparagus until tender-crisp.
2. Drizzle with olive oil, sprinkle with lemon zest, and season with salt and pepper for a vibrant side dish.

Mashed Sweet Potatoes

Ingredients:

- Sweet potatoes, peeled and cubed
- Low-sodium vegetable or chicken broth
- Olive oil or unsalted butter
- Herbs (optional)

Nutritional Information:

Calories	Protein	Carbohydrates	Fat
120	2g	25g	3g

Preparation:

1. Boil sweet potatoes until tender, then mash.
2. Add a small amount of low-sodium broth and olive oil or unsalted butter while mashing for a creamy texture.
3. Season with herbs, if desired.

Roasted Brussels Sprouts with Balsamic Glaze

Ingredients:

- Brussels sprouts, halved
- Olive oil
- Balsamic glaze (low-sodium)

Nutritional Information:

Calories	Protein	Carbohydrates	Fat
60	3g	10g	2g

Preparation:

1. Toss halved Brussels sprouts in olive oil and roast until tender and slightly browned.
2. Drizzle with low-sodium balsamic glaze for a tangy and nutritious side dish.

Sauteed Garlic Spinach

Ingredients:

- Fresh spinach leaves
- Minced garlic
- Olive oil
- Lemon juice (optional)

Nutritional Information:

Calories	Protein	Carbohydrates	Fat
40	3g	5g	2g

Preparation:

1. Sauté minced garlic in olive oil until fragrant.
2. Add fresh spinach and cook until wilted.
3. Finish with a squeeze of lemon juice for added freshness.

Cauliflower Rice Pilaf

Ingredients:

- Riced cauliflower
- Diced onions and bell peppers
- Low-sodium vegetable broth
- Herbs and spices (such as turmeric, cumin)

Nutritional Information:

Calories	Protein	Carbohydrates	Fat
50	3g	10g	2g

Preparation:

1. Sauté diced onions and bell peppers in a pan until tender.
2. Add riced cauliflower and cook until slightly softened.
3. Pour in low-sodium vegetable broth, add herbs and spices, and simmer until the liquid is absorbed.

Tomato Basil Salad

Ingredients:

- Sliced tomatoes
- Chopped fresh basil
- Olive oil and balsamic vinegar (low-sodium)

Nutritional Information:

Calories	Protein	Carbohydrates	Fat
70	2g	5g	5g

Preparation:

1. Arrange sliced tomatoes on a plate.
2. Sprinkle with chopped fresh basil and drizzle with a mixture of olive oil and low-sodium balsamic vinegar for a simple and flavorful salad.

Sautéed Green Beans with Almonds

Ingredients:

- Fresh green beans, trimmed
- Slivered almonds
- Olive oil
- Lemon zest (optional)

Nutritional Information:

Calories	Protein	Carbohydrates	Fat
70	3g	5g	5g

Preparation:

1. Sauté green beans in olive oil until tender.
2. Toast slivered almonds in a separate pan.
3. Toss green beans with toasted almonds and a sprinkle of lemon zest for a delightful side dish.

Guacamole

Ingredients:

- Ripe avocados, mashed
- Diced tomatoes and onions
- Chopped cilantro
- Lime juice
- Salt and pepper

Nutritional Information:

Calories	Protein	Carbohydrates	Fat
50	1g	3g	4g

Preparation:

1. In a bowl, combine mashed avocados, diced tomatoes, onions, and chopped cilantro.
2. Squeeze in fresh lime juice and season with salt and pepper.

3. Mix well and serve as a delicious dip for vegetables or whole-grain chips.

Salsa Fresca

Ingredients:

- Diced tomatoes
- Diced onions
- Chopped cilantro
- Minced jalapeño (optional for heat)
- Lime juice
- Salt and pepper

Nutritional Information:

Calories	Protein	Carbohydrates	Fat
10	0.5g	2g	0g

Preparation:

1. Combine diced tomatoes, onions, cilantro, and minced jalapeño in a bowl.

2. Squeeze fresh lime juice over the mixture and season with salt and pepper.

3. Allow the flavors to meld for a while before serving as a tasty salsa for chips or as a condiment.

Black Bean Dip

Ingredients:

- Canned black beans (low-sodium), drained and rinsed
- Minced garlic
- Cumin
- Lime juice
- Olive oil

Nutritional Information:

Calories	Protein	Carbohydrates	Fat
30	1g	5g	1g

Preparation:

1. Blend black beans, minced garlic, cumin, lime juice, and a touch of olive oil in a food processor until smooth.
2. Adjust seasonings to taste and serve as a protein-rich dip for vegetables or whole-grain crackers.

Low-Sodium Hummus

Ingredients:

- Cooked chickpeas, drained
- Tahini (sesame seed paste)
- Lemon juice
- Minced garlic
- Olive oil

Nutritional Information:

Calories	Protein	Carbohydrates	Fat
40	2g	5g	2g

Preparation:

1. Blend cooked chickpeas, tahini, lemon juice, minced garlic, and a drizzle of olive oil in a food processor until creamy.
2. Add a little water if needed for desired consistency and serve as a flavorful dip.

Cucumber Raita

Ingredients:

- Grated cucumber
- Low-fat Greek yogurt
- Chopped mint leaves
- Cumin
- Salt

Nutritional Information:

Calories	Protein	Carbohydrates	Fat
15	1g	2g	0g

Preparation:

1. Mix grated cucumber, low-fat Greek yogurt, chopped mint leaves, cumin, and a pinch of salt in a bowl.

2. Refrigerate before serving and enjoy this cooling dip with various dishes.

Roasted Red Pepper Dip

Ingredients:

- Roasted red peppers (from a jar), drained
- Plain low-fat yogurt or sour cream
- Minced garlic
- Paprika
- Olive oil

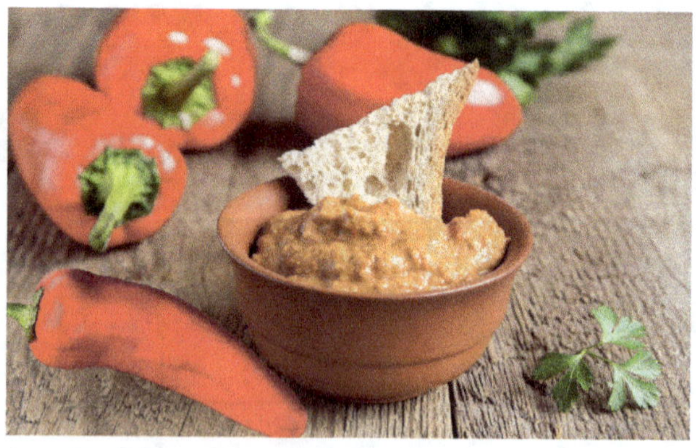

Nutritional Information:

Calories	Protein	Carbohydrates	Fat
30	1g	3g	2g

Preparation:

1. Blend roasted red peppers, plain low-fat yogurt or sour cream, minced garlic, paprika, and a drizzle of olive oil until smooth.

2. Serve this vibrant and tangy dip alongside fresh veggies or pita chips.

Tomato and Corn Salsa

Ingredients:

- Diced tomatoes
- Cooked corn kernels
- Chopped red onions
- Chopped cilantro
- Lime juice
- Salt and pepper

Nutritional Information:

Calories	Protein	Carbohydrates	Fat
15	1g	3g	0g

Preparation:

1. Combine diced tomatoes, cooked corn kernels, red onions, chopped cilantro, lime juice, salt, and pepper in a bowl.
2. Allow the flavors to meld before serving as a tasty salsa with grilled proteins or as a topping.

Greek Yogurt Dip with Herbs

Ingredients:

- Low-fat Greek yogurt
- Chopped dill and parsley
- Minced garlic
- Lemon juice
- Olive oil

Nutritional Information:

Calories	Protein	Carbohydrates	Fat
20	2g	2g	1g

Preparation:

1. Mix low-fat Greek yogurt with chopped dill, parsley, minced garlic, a squeeze of lemon juice, and a drizzle of olive oil.

2. Chill before serving with vegetable sticks or whole-grain pita for a refreshing dip.

3. These dips and sals

CHAPTER 6:

DESSERTS AND TREATS

Fruit-Based Sweets

Baked Apples

Ingredients:

- Apples (such as Granny Smith or Honeycrisp)
- Cinnamon
- Unsweetened apple juice or water
- Chopped nuts (optional)

Nutritional Information:

Calories	Protein	Carbohydrates	Fat
100	1g	25g	0.5g

Preparation:

1. Core the apples, leaving the bottom intact to hold the filling.

2. Sprinkle cinnamon inside each cored apple and place in a baking dish.

3. Pour unsweetened apple juice or water into the dish to prevent apples from drying out.

4. Bake at 350°F (175°C) for 30-40 minutes until tender. Optionally, top with chopped nuts.

Fruit Salad with Citrus Dressing

Ingredients:

- Assorted fresh fruits (such as berries, melon, grapes, and citrus segments)
- Lemon or orange juice
- Honey or sugar substitute (optional)

Nutritional Information:

Calories	Protein	Carbohydrates	Fat
70	1g	18g	0.5g

Preparation:

1. Cut assorted fruits into bite-sized pieces and combine in a bowl.

2. Mix fresh lemon or orange juice as a dressing. Add honey or sugar substitute if desired.

3. Toss the fruit salad in the citrus dressing and refrigerate before serving.

Frozen Banana Bites

Ingredients:

- Bananas, sliced
- Unsweetened peanut or almond butter
- Chopped nuts or shredded coconut (optional)

Nutritional Information:

Calories	Protein	Carbohydrates	Fat
80	2g	10g	4g

Preparation:

1. Spread unsweetened nut butter on banana slices and sandwich them together.

2. Optionally, roll in chopped nuts or shredded coconut.

3. Freeze until firm for a delightful, creamy treat.

Berry Compote

Ingredients:

- Mixed berries (such as strawberries, blueberries, and raspberries)
- Lemon juice
- Sugar substitute (optional)

Nutritional Information:

Calories	Protein	Carbohydrates	Fat
30	0.5g	8g	0g

Preparation:

1. Combine mixed berries, a splash of lemon juice, and a sweetener (if desired) in a saucepan.
2. Simmer on low heat until the berries break down and form a sauce. Let it cool before serving.

Grilled Peaches with Honey

Ingredients:

- Ripe peaches, halved and pitted
- Honey or sugar substitute
- Cinnamon (optional)

Nutritional Information:

Calories	Protein	Carbohydrates	Fat
40	1g	10g	0g

Preparation:

1. Brush peach halves with honey or sugar substitute.

2. Grill for a few minutes on each side until grill marks form. Sprinkle with cinnamon if desired.

Pineapple Coconut Popsicles

Ingredients:

- Fresh pineapple chunks
- Coconut water or unsweetened coconut milk

Nutritional Information:

Calories	Protein	Carbohydrates	Fat
40	0.5g	10g	0.5g

Preparation:

1. Blend fresh pineapple chunks with 1 coconut water or unsweetened coconut milk until smooth.

2. Pour the mixture into popsicle molds and freeze until solid for a refreshing frozen dessert.

Mango Sorbet

Ingredients:

- Fresh or frozen mango chunks
- Lemon juice
- Sugar substitute (optional)

Nutritional Information:

Calories	Protein	Carbohydrates	Fat
60	1g	15g	0.5g

Preparation:

1. Blend mango chunks, lemon juice, and sweetener (if desired) until smooth.

2. Transfer the mixture into a shallow dish and freeze. Stir every 30 minutes for a few hours until a sorbet consistency forms.

Low-Phosphorus Desserts

Rice Pudding

Ingredients:

- Arborio rice
- Low-phosphorus milk or almond milk
- Sugar substitute
- Cinnamon
- Raisins (optional)

Nutritional Information:

Calories	Protein	Carbohydrates	Fat

150	4g	30g	1.5g

Preparation:

1. Cook arborio rice in low-phosphorus milk or almond milk with a sweetener and cinnamon until creamy.
2. Optionally, stir in raisins. Chill before serving for a comforting dessert.

Vanilla Panna Cotta

Ingredients:

- Unflavored gelatin
- Low-phosphorus milk or coconut milk
- Sugar substitute
- Vanilla extract

Nutritional Information:

Calories	Protein	Carbohydrates	Fat
100	5g	5g	1g

Preparation:

1. Dissolve unflavored gelatin in low-phosphorus milk over low heat.
2. Add a sweetener and vanilla extract. Pour into molds and refrigerate until set.

Coconut Chia Seed Pudding

Ingredients:

- Chia seeds
- Low-phosphorus coconut milk
- Sugar substitute
- Unsweetened shredded coconut

Nutritional Information:

Calories	Protein	Carbohydrates	Fat
120	3g	10g	8g

Preparation:

1. Mix chia seeds with low-phosphorus coconut milk and a sweetener in a bowl. Refrigerate overnight.
2. Sprinkle with unsweetened shredded coconut before serving.

Banana Ice Cream

Ingredients:

- Frozen bananas
- Low-phosphorus milk or almond milk
- Unsweetened cocoa powder (optional)
- Sugar substitute

Nutritional Information:

Calories	Protein	Carbohydrates	Fat
100	1.5g	25g	0.5g

Preparation:

1. Blend frozen bananas with low-phosphorus milk until creamy. Add cocoa powder for chocolate flavor if desired.

2. Sweeten to taste, then freeze until firm for a healthy, creamy dessert.

Berry Parfait

Ingredients:

- Mixed berries (such as strawberries, blueberries, raspberries)
- Low-phosphorus yogurt or Greek yogurt
- Sugar substitute
- Crushed low-phosphorus cookies (optional)

Nutritional Information:

Calories	Protein	Carbohydrates	Fat
120	5g	20g	1g

Preparation:

1. Layer mixed berries and low-phosphorus yogurt in a glass.

2. Optionally, sprinkle crushed low-phosphorus cookies between layers for added texture.

Apple Crisp

Ingredients:

- Sliced apples
- Cinnamon
- Oats
- Almond flour
- Sugar substitute

Nutritional Information:

Calories	Protein	Carbohydrates	Fat
130	2.5g	25g	2g

Preparation:

1. Mix sliced apples with cinnamon in a baking dish.
2. In a separate bowl, combine oats, almond flour, and a sweetener, then sprinkle over the apples.
3. Bake until the topping is golden and the apples are tender.

Sweet Beverage Alternatives

Iced Herbal Tea with Lemon and Honey

Ingredients:

- Herbal tea bags (such as chamomile or hibiscus)
- Water
- Fresh lemon slices
- Honey or sugar substitute

Nutritional Information:

Calories	Potassium	Carbohydrates	Fat

10	0mg	3g	0g

Preparation:

1. Steep herbal tea bags in hot water, then chill.
2. Add fresh lemon slices and sweeten with honey or a sugar substitute for a refreshing and low-calorie beverage.

Watermelon Lime Cooler

Ingredients:

- Fresh watermelon chunks
- Lime juice
- Water
- Sugar substitute

Nutritional Information:

Calories	Potassium	Carbohydrates	Fat
50	180mg	15g	0g

Preparation:

1. Blend fresh watermelon chunks with lime juice and water until smooth.

2. Sweeten with a sugar substitute if desired and serve over ice for a hydrating and delicious cooler.

Cranberry Spritzer

Ingredients:

- Unsweetened cranberry juice
- Sparkling water
- Lime wedges
- Sugar substitute

Nutritional Information:

Calories	Potassium	Carbohydrates	Fat
30	10mg	8g	0g

Preparation:

1. Mix unsweetened cranberry juice with sparkling water.
2. Squeeze lime wedges for extra flavor and add a sugar substitute if desired for a tart and fizzy beverage.

Iced Peach and Ginger Green Tea

Ingredients:

- Green tea bags
- Sliced peaches
- Fresh ginger slices
- Water
- Sugar substitute

Nutritional Information:

Calories	Potassium	Carbohydrates	Fat
20	60mg	5g	0g

Preparation:

1. Brew green tea with fresh peach slices and ginger.

2. Sweeten with a sugar substitute, chill, and serve over ice for a soothing and lightly flavored tea.

Minty Pineapple Refresher

Ingredients:

- Fresh pineapple chunks
- Fresh mint leaves
- Water
- Sugar substitute

Nutritional Information:

Calories	Potassium	Carbohydrates	Fat
30	80mg	8g	0g

Preparation:

1. Blend fresh pineapple chunks with mint leaves and water until smooth.

2. Sweeten with a sugar substitute and serve over ice for a tropical and refreshing drink.

Blueberry Lemonade

Ingredients:

- Fresh blueberries
- Fresh lemon juice
- Water
- Sugar substitute

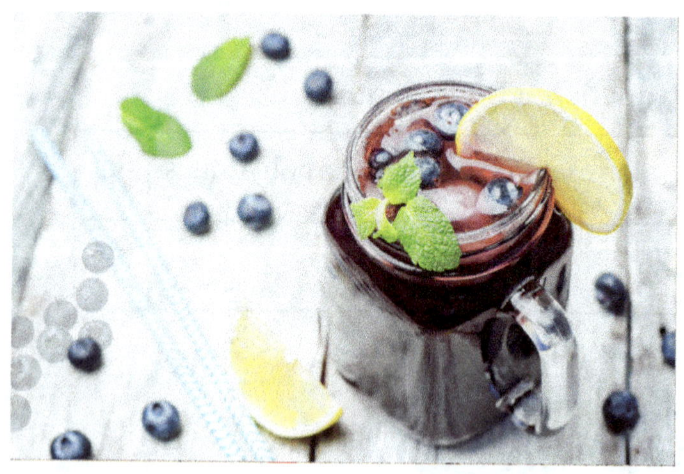

Nutritional Information:

Calories	Potassium	Carbohydrates	Fat
40	120mg	10g	0g

Preparation:

1. Blend fresh blueberries with lemon juice and water.
2. Add a sugar substitute, strain, and serve over ice for a tangy and delightful lemonade.

CHAPTER 7:

30 DAYS MEAL PLANS

Day 1:

Breakfast: Greek Yogurt Parfait

Snack: Baby Carrots

Lunch: Quinoa and Vegetable Salad

Snack: Apple Slices with Almond Butter

Dinner: Baked Salmon with Lemon and Dill

Day 2:

Breakfast: Oatmeal with Blueberries and Almonds

Snack: Mixed Berries

Lunch: Tuna Salad with Low-Sodium Dressing

Snack: Greek Yogurt

Dinner: Grilled Chicken Salad with Mixed Greens

Day 3:

Breakfast: Berry Smoothie

Snack: Cucumber Slices with Hummus

Lunch: Lentil and Vegetable Curry

Snack: Watermelon Chunks

Dinner: Vegetable and Chicken Kebabs

Day 4:

Breakfast: Quinoa Breakfast Bowl

Snack: Sliced Peppers with Greek Yogurt Dip

Lunch: Turkey and Avocado Wrap with Whole-Grain Tortilla

Snack: Mixed Nuts

Dinner: Grilled Shrimp with Lemon Garlic Sauce

Day 5:

Breakfast: Cottage Cheese and Peaches

Snack: Banana

Lunch: Roasted Red Pepper and Chickpea Salad

Snack: Cherry Tomatoes

Dinner: Turkey and Vegetable Stir-Fry

Day 6:

Breakfast: Rice Cake with Peanut Butter

Snack: Strawberries

Lunch: Homemade Low-Sodium Soup

Snack: Pineapple Slices

Dinner: Ratatouille with Herbs

Day 7:

Breakfast: Vegetable and Mushroom Omelette

Snack: Snap Peas

Lunch: Baked Pork Tenderloin with Herbs

Snack: Low-Sodium Popcorn

Dinner: Roast Beef and Swiss Cheese Sandwich on Whole-Grain Bread

Day 8:

Breakfast: Baked Lemon Herb Chicken

Snack: Sliced Cucumber with Tzatziki

Lunch: Quinoa and Black Bean Salad

Snack: Kiwi Slices

Dinner: Lemon Garlic Shrimp

Day 9:

Breakfast: Grilled Salmon with Dill Sauce

Snack: Edamame

Lunch: Roasted Vegetable and Feta Quiche

Snack: Melon Balls

Dinner: Chicken and Rice Soup

Day 10:

Breakfast: Vegetable Stir-Fry

Snack: Apple Slices

Lunch: Tofu and Vegetable Teriyaki Stir-Fry

Snack: Cherry Tomatoes

Dinner: Baked Zucchini and Tomato Casserole

Day 11:

Breakfast: Turkey and Vegetable Soup

Snack: Greek Yogurt with Honey

Lunch: Greek Salad with Low-Potassium Olives

Snack: Sliced Bell Peppers with Hummus

Dinner: Shrimp and Broccoli Alfredo with Low-Phosphorus Pasta

Day 12:

Breakfast: Spinach and Mushroom Stuffed Chicken

Snack: Berries

Lunch: Turkey Chili with Kidney-Friendly Beans

Snack: Baby Carrots

Dinner: Spinach and Feta Stuffed Chicken Breast

Day 13:

Breakfast: Lemon Herb Roasted Chicken Thighs

Snack: Mixed Nuts

Lunch: Chicken and Asparagus Stir-Fry

Snack: Watermelon Chunks

Dinner: Grilled Tofu with Pesto

Day 14:

Breakfast: Tofu and Vegetable Stir-Fry

Snack: Snap Peas

Lunch: Baked Sweet Potato and Black Bean Enchiladas

Snack: Mixed Berries

Dinner: Baked Chicken with Roasted Vegetables

Day 15:

Breakfast: Chili Lime Shrimp Tacos

Snack: Cucumber Slices with Greek Yogurt Dip

Lunch: Ratatouille with Herbs

Snack: Sliced Bell Peppers with Hummus

Dinner: Sesame Ginger Tofu and Broccoli

Day 16:

Breakfast: Vegetable and Chicken Kebabs

Snack: Baby Carrots

Lunch: Roasted Red Pepper and Chickpea Salad

Snack: Apple Slices with Almond Butter

Dinner: Grilled Pork Tenderloin with Herbs

Day 17:

Breakfast: Chicken and Rice Soup

Snack: Mixed Nuts

Lunch: Tofu and Vegetable Teriyaki Stir-Fry

Snack: Kiwi Slices

Dinner: Chicken and Asparagus Stir-Fry

Day 18:

Breakfast: Baked Zucchini and Tomato Casserole

Snack: Mixed Berries

Lunch: Roasted Vegetable and Feta Quiche

Snack: Watermelon Chunks

Dinner: Grilled Tofu with Pesto

Day 19:

Breakfast: Grilled Tofu with Pesto

Snack: Snap Peas

Lunch: Baked Sweet Potato and Black Bean Enchiladas

Snack: Cherry Tomatoes

Dinner: Baked Chicken with Roasted Vegetables

Day 20:

Breakfast: Baked Sweet Potato and Black Bean Enchiladas

Snack: Greek Yogurt with Honey

Lunch: Greek Salad with Low-Potassium Olives

Snack: Sliced Cucumber with Tzatziki

Dinner: Shrimp and Broccoli Alfredo with Low-Phosphorus Pasta

Day 21:

Breakfast: Ratatouille with Herbs

Snack: Edamame

Lunch: Turkey Chili with Kidney-Friendly Beans

Snack: Melon Balls

Dinner: Spinach and Feta Stuffed Chicken Breast

Day 22:

Breakfast: Baked Lemon Herb Chicken

Snack: Sliced Peppers with Hummus

Lunch: Quinoa and Black Bean Salad

Snack: Banana

Dinner: Lemon Garlic Shrimp

Day 23:

Breakfast: Grilled Salmon with Dill Sauce

Snack: Strawberries

Lunch: Roasted Vegetable and Feta Quiche

Snack: Low-Sodium Popcorn

Dinner: Roast Beef and Swiss Cheese Sandwich on Whole-Grain Bread

Day 24:

Breakfast: Tuna Salad with Low-Sodium Dressing

Snack: Baby Carrots

Lunch: Homemade Low-Sodium Soup

Snack: Pineapple Slices

Dinner: Ratatouille with Herbs

Day 25:

Breakfast: Turkey and Avocado Wrap with Whole-Grain Tortilla

Snack: Mixed Berries

Lunch: Tofu and Vegetable Teriyaki Stir-Fry

Snack: Watermelon Chunks

Dinner: Baked Zucchini and Tomato Casserole

Day 26:

Breakfast: Vegetable and Mushroom Omelette

Snack: Cucumber Slices with Greek Yogurt Dip

Lunch: Chicken and Rice Soup

Snack: Apple Slices with Almond Butter

Dinner: Grilled Chicken Salad with Mixed Greens

Day 27:

Breakfast: Rice Cake with Peanut Butter

Snack: Mixed Nuts

Lunch: Baked Salmon with Lemon and Dill

Snack: Kiwi Slices

Dinner: Baked Lemon Herb Chicken

Day 28:

Breakfast: Berry Smoothie

Snack: Snap Peas

Lunch: Cottage Cheese and Peaches

Snack: Cherry Tomatoes

Dinner: Grilled Salmon with Dill Sauce

Day 29:

Breakfast: Quinoa Breakfast Bowl

Snack: Greek Yogurt with Honey

Lunch: Vegetable and Mushroom Omelette

Snack: Sliced Bell Peppers with Hummus

Dinner: Tuna Salad with Low-Sodium Dressing

Day 30:

Breakfast: Greek Yogurt Parfait

Snack: Baby Carrots

Lunch: Quinoa and Vegetable Salad

Snack: Apple Slices with Almond Butter

Dinner: Baked Salmon with Lemon and Dill

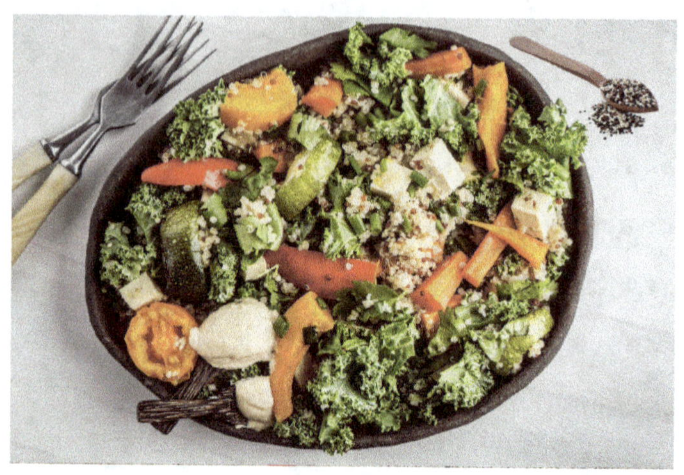

Your feedback is incredibly valuable. After exploring the "Renal Diet Cookbook for Beginners," your thoughts hold immense significance. Your review serves as a guiding light for those embarking on their kidney-healthy journey. Share how the recipes resonated with you and if the nutritional insights supported your understanding of kidney health. Your insights pave the way for future readers, aiding them in making informed choices and finding the right resources. Your thoughts illuminate the strengths and help in refining the book for future editions, ensuring it remains an indispensable tool for others seeking a healthier lifestyle. Your experiences are not just appreciated but cherished, as they inspire and support fellow readers in their quest for improved well-being. Please take a moment to share your thoughts and be a beacon for others on a similar path.

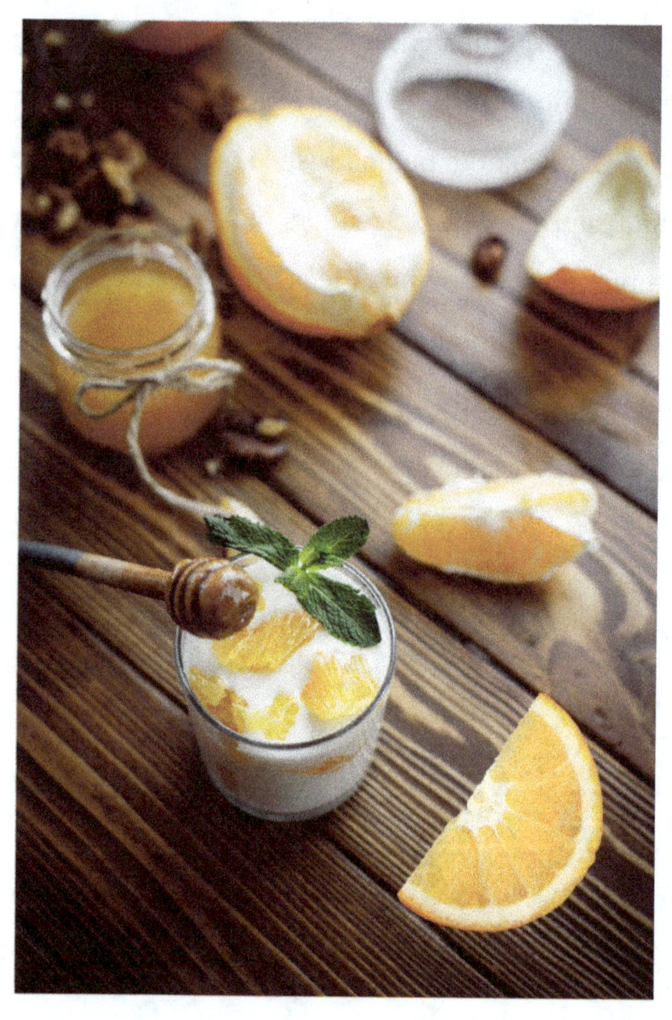

CHAPTER 8:

CONCLUSION

Embracing a Kidney-Healthy Diet

Embracing a kidney-healthy diet is not just a dietary choice; it's a pathway to nurturing your overall well-being. A kidney-healthy diet is a carefully curated approach that focuses on maintaining the optimal function of the kidneys, essential organs responsible for filtering waste and toxins from the body. It's a lifestyle centered around consuming the right balance of nutrients while managing the intake of substances that can burden these vital organs.

This dietary path involves embracing whole, unprocessed foods, emphasizing fruits, vegetables, lean proteins, and whole grains while moderating the intake of sodium, potassium, and phosphorus. Such a diet is fundamental in regulating blood pressure, reducing stress on the kidneys, and managing conditions like hypertension and diabetes, which are common culprits in kidney impairment. With a kidney-healthy diet, individuals can curate flavorsome meals rich in essential nutrients and flavors while adhering to the restrictions necessitated by renal health.

Choosing a kidney-healthy diet is not just a means to support the kidneys but also a way to promote vitality and improve one's quality of life. It involves making informed, health-conscious choices, fostering a mindful relationship with food, and valuing the remarkable impact of nutrition on the body's resilience. By embracing a kidney-healthy diet, individuals take an empowering step toward better health, vitality, and overall well-being.

Final Thoughts and Encouragement

In embarking on the journey of a renal diet, remember that each step, each recipe, and every mindful choice you make holds immense value in your overall well-being. A renal diet isn't just a list of foods to eat or avoid; it's a means of embracing a lifestyle that nurtures and supports your body's vitality.

As you explore the pages of this renal diet cookbook for beginners, may you discover a world of flavors, textures, and innovative culinary experiences that align with your health goals. Remember, this journey isn't about restriction; it's about adaptation and exploration. It's an invitation to get creative, to embrace new ingredients, and to craft dishes that delight your taste buds while honoring the needs of your body.

It's okay to take your time, to seek support, and to celebrate each small victory along the way. Embrace the learning curve, listen to your body, and celebrate the positive changes you're making for your health. Know that each meal prepared with care and each choice made mindfully is a step towards enhancing your well-being.

Above all, be kind to yourself. The path to a healthier lifestyle is a journey of self-care, self-discovery, and ultimately, self-empowerment. By choosing this path, you are taking a remarkable step towards better health and a more vibrant life. Stay curious, stay determined, and most importantly, stay encouraged on this invaluable journey towards wellness.

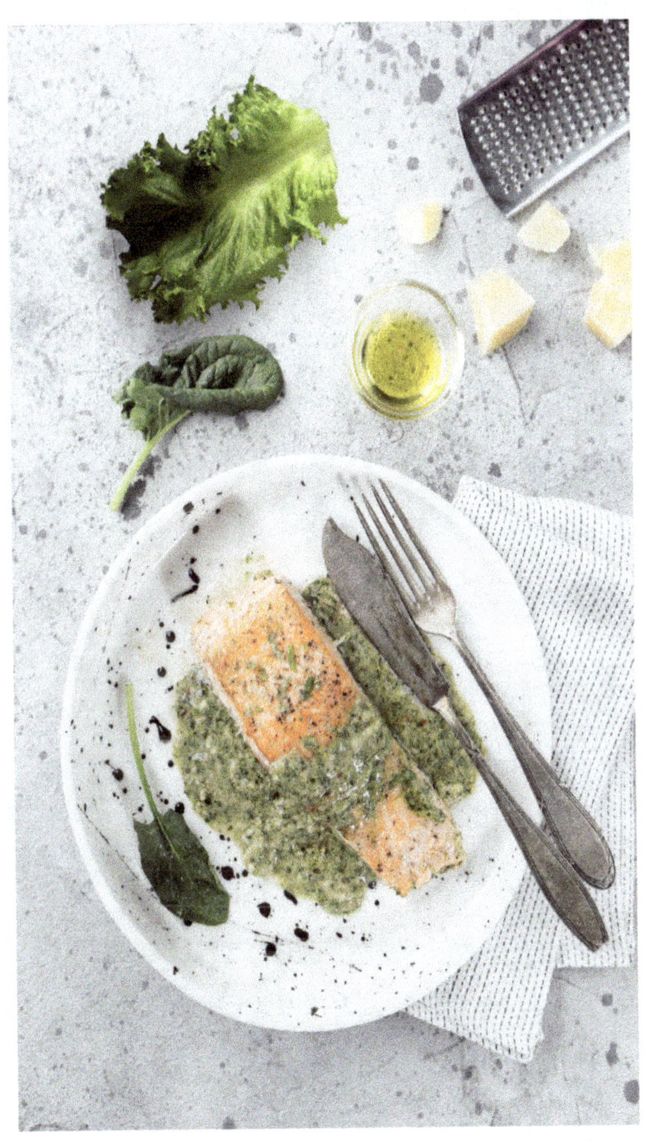

www.ingramcontent.com/pod-product-compliance
Lightning Source LLC
Chambersburg PA
CBHW050815260726
48660CB00004B/1448